1 MONTH OF
FREE
READING

at
www.ForgottenBooks.com

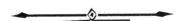

By purchasing this book you are
eligible for one month membership to
ForgottenBooks.com, giving you
unlimited access to our entire
collection of over 1,000,000 titles via
our web site and mobile apps.

To claim your free month visit:
www.forgottenbooks.com/free857175

ISBN 978-0-483-82528-4
PIBN 10857175

Dental Clippings.

ESTABLISHED NOVEMBER. 1898.

VOL. IV.	HOUSTON, TEXAS, JULY, 1902.	No. 9.

Logan and Amalgam Crowns.*

BY DR. B. F. BRUCE, ST. MATTHEWS, S. C.

I believe it has been said, that one of the earliest methods of loosening a tooth previous to extracting, was to tie a ligature around the neck, close to the cervical margin, and allow it opportunity to force its way up under the gum and render extraction less painful.

What would be the comment of our fellow practitioner, if such a method was employed at this time? It has been remarked, that the mistake of the physiican can be buried under the ground; fittingly true; the dentist can bury his ill-fitting gold bands beneath the gnms, only to be safe for a season.

Thus, rather than proving a benefit, the result is often a positive detriment to the tooth, as well as to the general health.

It cannot be gainsaid, that when an all banded crown is removed after a few years service, it is so foul from accumulation of food particles, that one's stomach revolts from the nauseating odor. For illustration, ream out the cement of the gold crown that has been broken off, and notice the unbearable odor evolving from the burring.

Of course, this condition only exists where the crown or band is not properly fitted; but the majority of the so-called shell or banded crowns, have been improperly fitted.

Notice if you please, the very nature of the operation, and compare that class of work with that of the Logan crown, for the teeth anterior to the molars, and the amalgam crown, for the molar teeth, and I think you will find the Logan and amalgam crowns to be far superior to banded crowns.

For instance, take a superior lateral insisor. Cut it off, leaving a portion of the enamel on the lingual side, and passing on

*Read before the South Carolina State Dental Association.

CONTENTS FOR FEBRUARY, 1902.

Page

ORIGINAL CONTRIBUTION—

Facial Neuralgia, as Observed by the Busy Dentist, by Dr. C. E. FRAZER, Weatherford, Texas.. 65— 69

On the Management of the Permanent Superior Incisors and Bicuspids, by D. L. G. NOEL, D. D. S., Nashville, Tenn.. 69— 75

Putty as a Root Filling .... 75— 78

Ethical Advertising... 78— 79

Dentistry as a Profession. .... 79— 80

In the Attic, by GUSTAVE P. WICKSELL.. 80— 82

Smoking and Epithelioma of the Tongue... 82— 83

Decision of Judge Townsend in the Kyle Case.................................... 83— 84

To Remove Pulp under Pressure Anæsthesia...................................... 84

EDITORIAL DEPARTMENT—

Items 85

The Texas State Dental Association... 85

Patents Relating to Dentistry.. 86— 87

Advertisements.. I—XVII

Dental Clippings.

ESTABLISHED NOVEMBER, 1898.

VOL. IV. HOUSTON, TEXAS, JUNE, 1902. No. 8.

Original Contributions.

On the Use of Psycratism in Dental Surgery.

BY DR. J. S. M'DONALD, D. D. S., AND PROFESSOR OF PSYCRATISM,
ZACATECAS, MEXICO.

Psychratism, as a term, is eminently proper for the science generally known as mesmerism, hypnotism, etc., deriving the word from the Greek roots "psychos" (mind, or soul) and "kratos" (prowess, superior power, power over, force, or mastery). Joining these two words, we have "psychratism," as the last syllable of the first root and the first one of the second are of the same sound, and it is permissible to join the two by running these two into one and thus making a euphonious whole, the "ism" meaning a condition, according to Professor Vernon, who coined the word, and from whom I am indebted for the little I know about the science. Having explained the meaning of the word or term, I will now go into the science a little deeper and explain where it may be useful in dentistry as an anesthetic in minor surgery. Every operator knows from experience that suggestion is very important. To those who have not thought about it before, allow me to explain more fully: Suppose a person comes into your office to have a tooth extracted. There are two classes. The majority confesses that the pain ceased as soon as they reached your door, which demonstrates that they could put their mind upon something else besides the aching tooth. In those cases you can employ psychratism; in other words, you can impress them with a suggestion, providing you can draw their minds away from the idea that you are going to hurt them, and impress them with the idea that they will not suffer. About the other class (happily the minority), where the aching tooth will not allow them

A Legal Identification.*

BY E. S. ROSENBLUTH, D.D.S., BRIDGEPORT, CONN.

A murder trial hinging largely upon the expert testimony of a dentist is quite uncommon. This fact being conceded, I have been persuaded to relate my experience in connection with the trial of the midwife, Nancy A. Guilford, who was accused of murder as the result of a criminal operation which caused the death of a young woman, named Emma Gill, a resident of Southington, Conn., where I was then located. I confess to a certain degree of reluctance in taking up this subject, and do so only because I have been urged, on the ground that it is of general interest to the profession.

Early in September, 1898, several dismembered portions of a female human body were found on the water front of Bridgeport, Conn., near what is known as the Yellow Mill Pond bridge. The fact that a large number of young women were then missing from their homes in this State, as well as in Massachusetts, caused many interested relatives to view the remains, as yet lying unidentified at an undertaking establishment in Bridgeport, which served as a morgue.

The father of a young woman resident in a small town in Massachusetts, who came to view the body, was satisfied that it was that of his daughter; and with the assurance of his family dentist, who had not examined the teeth, but reached his conclusions from a description of them, the body was delivered to the family for burial. Upon arrival at his home the father was amazed to find that his daughter had returned alive and well. The body, therefore, was returned to the morgue in Bridgeport.

About this time it became known that a young woman, named Emma Gill, was missing from Southington, Conn. The local correspondent of the *Hartford Courant* was the first to surmise the true identity of the corpse, and upon seeing the head, which had been severed from the body, he concluded that it bore a striking resemblance to that young woman. He requested several members of her family to view the remains, which they did, with the result that the father, three brothers, and a sister confirmed him in his belief.

It being known to her parents that their daughter had been one of my patients, they so informed the chief of police of Bridgeport, who thereupon called me by telephone, requesting

*Read before the Hartford, Conn., Dental Society, January 13, 1902.

that I come there at once and make an examination of the mouth. Having a full appointment-book, and no curiosity whatever, I declined to do so, on the ground that professional engagements demanded all my time. I, however, sent him a chart showing the condition of the teeth of Emma Gill, so that it could be used for purposes of comparison should he desire an examination of the head by a local dentist.

An examination was at once ordered, and was made, the findings being presented at the inquest by Dr. G. C. Eighm, of Bridgeport, whose chart, upon comparison, agreed with mine. This satisfied the authorities, and the body was surrendered to the Gill family, who removed it to Southington for burial.

It was, of course, known that a crime had been committed, but by whom was still unknown. The police authorities were at work on the case, and it was gradually developed that a midwife, Mrs. Guilford, of Bridgeport, was connected with the case, and it was further found that others had assisted her in disposing of the body. The arrests of Mrs. Guilford, her son, her daughter, and a colored maid followed. Evidence was rapidly accumulating, and a prosecution for murder in the second degree determined upon by the State's attorney of the district.

The body was then in Southington for interment. As the funeral procession was passing my office, Coroner Doten, of Bridgeport, called me by telephone and requested that I make a careful examination of the teeth; it was, however, too late, and I so informed him. The following morning I received a telegram from the coroner, reiterating his request, and saying that the State would pay for the service. Detectives Arnold and Cronin, of the Bridgeport police force, called at my office soon after the receipt of this telegram, relating the coroner's purpose, and we agreed upon a time to disinter the body. Upon my suggestion, the detectives secured the services of an undertaker and a sexton. They also procured a permit for the disinterment.

The head only was removed from the grave, and was conveyed to what is known as the "tool-house" of the cemetery, a small wooden structure, containing no furniture excepting one broken chair, which was placed in the doorway to serve as a support for the head.

In the presence of the detectives, a local deputy sheriff, and others as witnesses, the examination was carefully conducted, with the knowledge that it was to be used in a court of justice for the prosecution of a criminal charge. It is, consequently, unnecessary to state that it was carefully performed, with the aid of Dr. W. G. Steadman, the health officer of the town, who noted in writing the progress of examination. I examined the mouth three times with exactly the same result.

The method employed was simple, a common cork being used to prop the jaws apart on one side, while the teeth on the other side were being examined with exploring instruments and a mouth mirror. Each filling was noted in detail, as to position, filling material used, and as nearly as possible the methods employed by the operator in finishing gold and amalgâm, the condition of the fillings and discoloration of materials from various causes. The head having been in sea-water, and subsequently placed in a jar of embalming fluid, a scum covered some of the amalgam fillings, which gave them the appearance of cement, deceiving those who saw the head in the morgue at Bridgeport. Missing teeth were noted, as well as decayed roots which remained.

Upon returning to my office, I made a careful transcript of my records of work done at the various sittings of Emma Gill, also of teeth which I had extracted for her, and found that the complete record was the same as the result of my examination of the head, excepting that my book indicated the extraction of the lower right first molar, and a later entry showed a filling in the same tooth, which was evidently contradictory, due, I felt satisfied, to a clerical error in my record. At any rate, the examination of the work found in the mouth examined revealed all the characteristic features of my methods of operating, all of which soon convinced me that the head examined at the cemetery could be none other than that of Emma Gill.

After an interval of about six months, the case was to be called in the Superior Court at Bridgeport, Judge George H. Wheeler, presiding. Not having received any notice that I would be called upon as a witness, but believing that it could not be avoided, I wrote to the Hon. Samuel Fessenden, the State's attorney for the district, inquiring as to his intentions, and requesting that, if possible, he leave me out of the case, since my practice demanded all of my time, and that I could not well afford to appear in court for sixty cents per day, the usual witness fee. He replied, requesting me to call on him at the Superior Court Building in Bridgeport, at a given time, which I did, and again reminded him of the fact that it would be decidedly unfair to claim my services, which he could do, at the ordinary witness fee. He, therefore, agreed that my bill for services should be taxed with the other costs of the case, and the next day confirmed this by letter.

When the case was called, I was summoned to appear in court at the very beginning of the trial. Thus many others, as well as myself, were required to sit quietly listening to the proceedings of organizing the jury and the testimony of other witnesses. At first it seemed like time wasted, but before much time had elapsed it dawned upon me that it was quite an advantage to grow accustomed to the surroundings, and especially to the methods employed in cross-examination by counsel for the defense. It was, of course, necessary that the prosecuting attorney establish the identity of the body, which he sought to do through the testimony of relatives and friends of the dead woman, as well as through the dental work found in the mouth.

Upon being called upon the witness stand, Mr. Fessenden at once sought to establish this fact, by bringing out the result of my examination of the mouth, with the transcript of my record-book, which was presented in detail.

There was no room for doubt, in my mind in relation to the identity of the dead woman, and I so testified in the most positive terms, although I had made no effort to recognize the features.

The Hillischer method, which I have employed since 1894 in recording my work, is simple, but quite positive, consisting of an entry in an ordinary journal stating the work performed and designating the position in the mouth of teeth filled, crowned, extracted, treated, or otherwise operated upon, by numbering from one to eight, and using a long, horizontal line crossed in the center. All figures above the line represent the upper teeth, and those below, the lower teeth. The crossed line stands for the median line of the mouth. To the right of the center or crossed line represents the right side of the mouth, and to the left, the left side of the mouth.

EXAMPLE:

$$\frac{8\text{-}7\text{-}6\text{-}5\text{-}4\text{-}3\text{-}2\text{-}1 \quad | \quad 1\text{-}2\text{-}3\text{-}4\text{-}5\text{-}6\text{-}7\text{-}8}{8\text{-}7\text{-}6\text{-}5\text{-}4\text{-}3\text{-}2\text{-}1 \quad | \quad 1\text{-}2\text{-}3\text{-}4\text{-}5\text{-}6\text{-}7\text{-}8}$$

The various surfaces of the teeth are designated by abbreviations, thus: M for mesial, D for distal, OC for occlusal, INC for incisal, AP for anterior pit, DP for distal pit, BU for buccal, LI for lingual, and so on.

Upon being turned over to the tender mercies of the defense for cross-examination, I immediately discovered that counsel for the defendant required that I qualify professionally. After giving my name and address, etc., the first technical question aimed at me was: "What is a tooth?" It came so unexpectedly that for a moment I could not give the technical definition without stopping to consider, so the best that I could do was to answer that it was of no consequence, as everybody knows what a tooth is.

The defendant's counsel, Mr. Klein, then examined me carefully in dental anatomy, the composition of various amalgam alloys, dental cements, bacteriology, and operative dentistry, in which he had probably been coached by a dental friend. He was quite creditably prepared. The differences between the crowns of the various upper and lower teeth interested him considerably.

It soon became apparent that a tooth not present in the head should be referred to, not as one extracted, but as missing.

An attempt was made to compel me to testify in relation to the location of fillings without my records before me. This I refused to do, on the ground that it was impossible to remember such details on the spur of the moment.

Having asserted that there is much individuality exhibited in the work of most operators, I was called upon to explain what there was peculiar about the work found in the severed head that I could identify as mine.

At that time I was in the habit of wafering amalgam for the finishing of such fillings, and when quite hard using a small ball burnisher, drawing it from the center to the edges, leaving no perceptible marks except upon the buccal surface, where there is little attrition to obliterate them.

There was such a filling on the buccal surface of the lower right first molar, which was the tooth involved in my clerical error, a filling recently made, with the radiating marks perceptible, which is quite unusual.

This was the cause of the following questioning:

Q. "Is there any difference in your work from the work of other dentists?"

A. "Yes. Dentists show individuality in their work."

Q. "What peculiarities had you?"

A. "The peculiarity of burnishing from the center to the edges of a filling."

Q. "If your burnisher is perfectly flat and larger than the cavity, would it be good dentistry to use it?"

A. "Yes, in some cases."

Q. "What was the size of the round burnisher that you used in this particular work?"

A. "I will not attempt to give such a measurement without the assistance of a standard gauge, but will bring it here with several others if you wish to examine it."

Q. "A flat burnisher is sometimes round, is it not?"

A. "A flat burnisher is flat."

The court here adjourned until the following Monday morning. In the meantime counsel for the defense was busily engaged in preparing several neatly laid traps, in which to entangle his witness, as will be seen later. I also was engaged in preparing an ocular demonstration for the benefit of counsel for the defense, in the shape of a series of amalgam fillings made in a tooth-brush handle, showing five or six methods of finishing such fillings.

On Monday morning I took an early train in order to present this to the State's attorney for his inspection. I also produced a handful of burnishers, including those of the small ball variety, all of which seemed to please him, and he said that he would call for them at the proper time. At 10 a. m. court convened promptly, and I was at once recalled to the witness-stand.

Counsel for the defense immediately proceeded to cross-examine me. I was now without my records to refer to, a dangerous situation, to which I demurred, but the court ruled that I must answer.

Q. "Why did you cap lower right number six?"

A. "I did not."

Q. "Did you find any fillings in the lower central incisors?"

A. "No."

Q. "Are you sure of it?"

A. "Certainly, I was very careful to note exactly the condition of the mouth I examined, as well as in keeping my records."

Q. "I know that you have said that before, but you did not notice the projection of an amalgam filling, did you?"

(The State's attorney entered an objection. Not sustained.)

A. "No one has testified that such a filling projected,

although one of the gold fillings appeared to have been disturbed by the point of a sharp instrument.''

After several more attempts of the same nature, which met with no better success, my record-book, together with the transcript of it which had thus far been used, was admitted in evidence. It now became necessary to prove the clerical error in my record-book, which was done to the satisfaction of the court and counsel. It was also necessary to swear that these records were entered on the same day on which the work was done, which, happily, I could do.

Mr. Fessenden called for the ivory tooth-brush handle, which I had prepared to demonstrate the various methods of finishing amalgam fillings, and requested me to mark the one that was burnished from the center to the edges, which I did, and he then offered it as an exhibit.

Counsel for the defense both fiercely objected to its admission, but the court ruled otherwise, and it was marked for identification. Mr. Fessenden then called for the ball burnisher in question, and after many objections this was also admitted and marked for identification. This practically ended my examination, and I was much pleased to note that the customary challenge against the admission of this line of testimony was not forthcoming.

The case proceeded from this point for about three weeks, during which much direct as well as expert medical testimony, in regard to malpractice, length of the dismembered body in life, etc., were taken, nearly all bearing heavily upon the guilt of the accused. The trial, however, came to a sudden halt, caused by the illness of one of the jurors, with little prospect for his early recovery.

After several days of waiting, the court reluctantly decided to dismiss the jury and order a new trial. The defense evidently having little hope of an acquittal, offered to plead guilty to manslaughter in the first degree, with the proviso that the cases against her children and colored maid be dropped. This compromise was accepted by the State, and the prisoner is now serving a sentence of ten years in Wethersfield prison.— *Dental Cosmos.*

Chloroform Claims Another Victim.

A sad accident, for accident it was, occured at the office of Dr. James A. Sampsell, New Orleans, La., on September 11th, whereby Mrs Mattie Glover, a young widow of only 24 years, lost her life.

The administration of chloroform is often attended by more or less danger, and the deadly drug is most insidious and uncertain in its effects. It has been known for many years—in fact, ever since the use of chloroform as an anesthetic became general—that persons subject to weakness of any of the vital organs, especially the heart, were endangered by its use, and physicians and surgeons, as well as dentists, are most careful in its administration. The latter rarely ever administer it unless a physician is present, yet even then deaths have been known to occur from its use. In the case yesterday the subject was in perfect health, and had been carefully examined prior to taking chloroform. Yet death overtook her even in the presence of her family physician, who was well acquainted with her system and had taken every precaution which science and skill could suggest to prevent an accident such as did occur through no fault of his. He had no reason to fear any bad results from the drug; in fact, to all intents and purposes, the lady was in no danger whatsoever from taking chloroform.

Dr. Joseph O'Hara was her family physician, and on Wednesday last Mrs. Glover notified him that she was going to have five teeth extracted and that she desired him to be present at the operation. Dr. O'Hara replied that he would be present at 11 o'clock. Mrs. Glover resided at No. 2512 Canal, near Rocheblave street, with an aunt, Mrs. William Hamblet, and she had requested Mrs. Kate Onion, a daughter-in-law of Captain Onion and also an aunt, to accompany her to Dr. Sampsell's office. Promptly at 11 o'clock the ladies entered the elevator and proceeded to the dentist's office. Dr. Sampsell was in, but Dr. O'Hara had not yet arrived, and while waiting for him the ladies engaged in conversation with Dr. Sampsell and Mr. Underwood, who has an office just in the rear of Dr. Sampsell's office. Presently Dr. O'Hara arrived, and Mrs. Glover prepared herself for the operation, divesting herself of her hat, and arranging her hair so that it would not occasion her any discomfort. She was seated in the dentist's chair, which can be raised or lowered to place the patient in any position the operator might desire. Dr. O'Hara made a cursory examination of the patient, not deeming it necessary to make a minute examination as to the condition of her heart, lungs, kidneys, etc., having made such an examination not long since. He felt her pulse and found it normal, and aside from the nervousness which any one would experience when having a tooth extracted, Mrs. Glover gave no indication of suffering at all. Dr. O'Hara administered the chloroform, and the first tooth was extracted and the patient immediately revived. Another small quantity of chloroform was administered and the second tooth was drawn, and the lady revived and spoke a few words to those who stood around her. A cork had been placed in her mouth to hold the jaws apart while she was under the influence of the drug, to faciliate the dentist in his work. Again the chloroform was administered and the third tooth was drawn, and then the fourth tooth was jerked out by the operator. Thus far all had gone well, and the patient exhibted no outward signs of being any the worse either from the drug or the shock of having the teeth drawn. While the last tooth was drawn, however, Mrs. Glover had bitten the cork in half, and Dr. O'Hara advised her to spit it out. She leaned over the side of the operating chair and expectorated and remarked quite pleasantly: "There's the cork," as it fell into the cupsidor. Turning to Mrs. Onion, Mrs. Glover asked, with a smile: "Did I cut up any?" Dr. O'Hara answered for Mrs. Onion, saying: "Oh, no; you did not. You did very nicely, indeed." Mrs. Onion then said: "Oh hurry up, and let's get through with this horrible job," for it is always more painful to witness the extraction of teeth than even to have them extracted. Mrs. Glover again laid back in a recumbent position, the chair having been gauged accordingly. Dr. O'Hara again administered the drug, and Mrs. Glover dropped off into unconsciousness. Dr. Sampsell pushed Dr. O'Hara's hand aside in order to introduce the forceps into the lady's mouth, but was unable to do so.

The last tooth was one of the molars, far back in the mouth, and he was unable to reach it. "She will have to sit up higher." said the dentist, and pressing on the spring which held the seat in position, he raised the patient's head slowly. Dr. O'Hara was watching her closely, when, to his horror, he saw the pupils of her eyes dilate and roll up under the lids. At once he became aware of the danger, and called hurriedly to Dr. Sampsell to lower the chair. Dr. Sampsell becoming excited, attempted to do so, but either he was too flurried to operate the chair, or the mechanism became deranged, but at any rate he could not move it. Immediately there was consternation in the room, Mrs. Onion became aware that something was amiss, and peered over the shoulders of the two doctors, but she could not conceive at the moment the true state of affairs. Dr. O'Hara, finding that the chair could not be lowered, and aware that every second was precious, picked the unconscious lady up and laid her on the floor. Then he commenced moving her arms up and down and in and out, in order to induce artificial respiration, Mrs. Onion lending all the assistance in her power. Meantime Mr. Underwood had heard the unusual noise in the room and came rushing in, and found Dr. O'Hara at work on the inanimate body. "Can I help you?" he asked. "No," responded Dr. O'Hara, "except you go as quickly as you can for a physician." Mr. Underwood sprang away from the party and hastened to the office of the State Board of Health, where he found Dr. Arthur Nolte. Hastily he told him of the accident, and of Dr. O'Hara's request, and Dr. Nolte went to the office of Dr. Sampsell. He found Dr. O'Hara still striving to induce respiration, and then suggested that stimulants be administered. Dr. O'Hara had already bethought himself of this, and had produced his hypodermic for that purpose. Meantime Dr. Nolte had placed his hand over the lady's heart, and just as Dr. O'Hara was about to administer the stimulant, Dr. Nolte stopped him with the sad words, "It's too late, doctor, she's dead."

Up to this time Mrs. Onion had controlled herself admirably, and had lent all the assistance in her power, but when Dr. Nolte spoke the fatal words she collapsed entirely and sank unconscious to the floor beside the corpse of her niece. When she recovered consciousness the baleful sight of the corpse of her loved relative met her view once more, and she became hysterical, and it was with the greatest difficulty that she could finally be calmed. Consternation reigned among the physicians, who gave no thought to anything else than to resuscitate the dead woman, even though they knew that their efforts would prove futile. For a long time they worked, but finally, in despair, abandoned the effort, and there was nothing left to do but to notify the coroner.

Dr. Richard responded promptly. He viewed the body, and after obtaining a statement of how the accident had occurred, he advised the removal of the body to the residence of the deceased, where he would hold an autopsy. Mr. B. B. Howard, an attorney, and a friend of the parties, Drs. Sampsell and O'Hara, accompanied the body to No. 2512 Canal street. Dr.

Richard had determined to hold an autopsy in order to ascertain beyond doubt the condition of the heart, lungs and kidneys, so that he might be able to attach any blame should any blame be attached to any one. The autopsy was held and the coroner found that death had been caused by anaemia of the brain, in other words, the blood had all left the brain and had flowed downward into the body, and this is what caused death. All the vital organs were found to be in perfect condition, the heart, the lungs, the liver, and the kidneys. It was obvious, therefore, that when the poor woman was raised up in the chair in order that Dr. Sampsell might reach the tooth which he was endeavoring to extract, the blood rushed downward into her system, leaving the brain bloodless, which was fully demonstrated and revealed by the autopsy.

Thoughts of the Profession.

BY DR. W. H. STEELE, HASTINGS, NEB.

I might have selected for my subject something more practical, and that would have called forth an interesting discussion from the intelligent members of the profession here assembled; but leaving those subjects for others better prepared to handle them, I shall bring up a few points bearing more directly on the business side of our profession.

Very few young men, when locating in a new town, realize how their every act from the furnishing of the new office, to the collection and paying of their bills, is watched and weighed, by an ever-observing, critical public. When a patient steps into our office for the first time an impression is usually formed for, or against us, and a tidy office has much more to do with the forming of this first impression and our future success, than we have any idea of. Our patients are more observing than we sometimes suppose, and notice things that reflect unfavorably upon us, hence, we need to be continually on the alert, and see that ourselves, our office appointments and instruments are such as will bear scrutiny and defy criticism. One may not be so financially situated that he can furnish an office elegantly, but there is no excuse for dusty furniture, unswept carpets, bespattered spittoons, and dirty instruments. A dentist who is particular about keeping his office and its appurtenances neat and orderly, is likely to be particular and thorough with his operations. The public know this, and it is a strong point in gaining public confidence and patronage. While a pleasant, well equipped office is a good introduction to a new patron, it requires much more than this to gain their confidence and respect and retain them. It demands integrity, cleanliness in all operations, thorough manipulation, artistic skill, kindness and courtesy. Many a good patient has been lost on account of a bloody spittoon, or a bill that had run so long that the charge was thought exorbitant when finally presented for payment. There is no profession in which the personality and artistic skill of the man cuts any more important figure than in dentistry, and the dentist possessing these qualities need not advertise his superiority through the press. His work gives every day unwritten evidence of his ability far more telling than anything that could be accomplished through the use of printer's ink, and its veracity cannot be questioned by the most skeptical. Too many dentists, especially in the early part of their career, make the mistake of relying too much on the distribution of printer's ink for the building up of their business. Let any enterprising, talented, incoming young member of the profession take the pains to instruct himself on the business methods of those dentists who have come out best, both financially and in reputation, after a twenty-five years' career, and see whether the successful men were those who relied on printer's ink. I think that he will find that those who have attained the greatest success are the ones whose aim has always been to do first-class work, work such as they might feel proud of, and at prices that remunerated them for the labor and skill which they bestowed upon it. Such methods require a little more time to build up a business, but they are sure to win the support they merit. The moral effect of a bank account on a man's business success cannot be overestimated. No man can do his best when his mind is distracted from his work. "Worry dries the blood more than care or sorrow," therefore it is essential, if a man would at all times be in a position to put forth his best efforts, that he be pecuniarily independent; that his finances and his credit be so perfectly established that a season of depression in business shall lose its terrors, and that worry at least from this source should be an unknown factor. It is easy to meet bills when business is good, but when poor it is a source of worry which affects the temper of the man and the quality of his work; he loses his feeling of independence, and unless he is an actor of more than moderate ability, this fact will soon become apparent to his patients. The only remedy for this evil is a bank account, that can be built up in good times and drawn upon when business is poor; by this means we will always be able to meet our patients with a smiling face and put forth our best efforts, instead of worrying about butchers' bills, tailors' bills and rents. Many bright young dentists who locate in the smaller towns are in danger of getting into a groove. They are fresh from school, up to date in methods, and soon get a good practice, but are liable to become avaricious and devote too much of their time to the business side of the profession. They do not keep read up, do not attend the dental societies, and about the time they should be at their best they are twenty years behind the times.

Young Dr. B.—— comes in and locates across the street; practice begins to drop off, and the old doctor awakens to the fact that he will have to move West and locate in a smaller town. We older members of the profession have all seen many such sad failures. The way to avoid it is to keep up with the times; take the dental journals; take an active part in your State and district societies, and thus avoid fossilization.—*Dental Review.*

Paraffin, an Ideal Material for the Filling of Root Canals.

We may attribute a large number of alveolar abscesses, failures of crowns, bridges and fillings, to imperfectly filled root canals. Considering the difficulty of following the irregular, tortuous and minute root canals, and the uncertainty as to the number of canals in some teeth, it is not remarkable that either portions or entire canals are left unfilled by the use of materials that are recommended, such as points of gutta-percha, gold, tin, lead, copper, wood or cotton, chlorid of zinc, cement, sandarac, etc.

The objection to these agents is that, their introduction into the roots is not certain to reach and hermetically seal the apical foramen so as to prevent the invasion of pathogenic micro organisms into the canals or apical space. Another objection is, that the cutting away of much tooth structure, especially in bicuspids and molars, is necessary in order to have sufficient space for the introduction of most of these materials, thus reducing the strength of the tooth.

In reading an article published by Pro.f R. Gersuny, of Vienna (*Zeitschrift fuer Heilkunde*, 1900, Vol. I, Pt. 9), in which he demonstrated that if paraffin at a low melting point be injected into the tissues of the body and allowed to harden, it will retain its solid consistency, remain there unchanged, and not be absorbed, the idea suggested itself to me that this same material could be utilized for the filling of root canals, and I at once set out to make experiments.

Permit me to submit the result of my experiments and the technique employed: A mixture of paraffin 96%, white vaselin 4%, is placed in a porcelain dish and brought to the boiling point; and if it be desired to color the same, alkanet may be added while being boiled. The tooth in which the roots are to be filled, after all the contents have been removed, is placed in an aseptic condition, and is thoroughly dried out with hot air.

I have employed two methods for the filling of root canals with paraffin: (1). By means of injection with Anal's metal syringe or Luer's glass syringe, which has been previously sterilized and kept warm, filled with liquid paraffin, inverted and all air expelled by pressing upon the piston. The needle is screwed firmly to the attachment and pressed again; the piston is to force the paraffin into the needle point. The charged syringe is placed in hot water until ready for use, in order to keep the paraffin in a liquid state. The root being ready for filling, the solution, which should be at a temperature of about 160° F., is injected into the tooth. It will readily flow to the desired points, where it shortly after becomes cooled and hard, and remains so. In filling roots of the upper denture, the patient is placed in a reclining position, or with head hanging. A heavy tin foil, or a lead disc with a central perforation, is placed over the orifice of the tooth, thus preventing the material from escaping. A straight point with the syringe is used. While filling the lower teeth the patient sits upright and a curved point is required.

The other method is, to my mind, preferable, especially in the lower denture. The roots are prepared in the same manner. A sufficient quanity of the mixed paraffine (previously boiled and allowed to harden, and kept sterile) to fill the number of roots is placed into the tooth. A soft metal disc with a central perforation is placed over the orifice of the tooth, and a continuous stream of hot air conducted from an apparatus devised by Dr. J. C. Beck, of Chicago, will dissolve and force the paraffin into every minute opening in the tooth. It is then allowed to cool and harden. I have employed the method with the material described in a large number of root fillings for the past twelve months with good results.

Conclusions.—(1). That the material can be made absolutely sterile by boiling. (2). Readily adapted to the walls of the space it is designed to fill, and unchanged by the influences of the body. (3). Not necessary to cut away as much tooth structure for its insertion. (4). Less time to insert, and especially to remove. (5). Absolutely painless to the patient while being inserted, and no tenderness of the tooth, which is so frequently mentioned, after the roots are filled.

In this connection I desire to point out another utility of the mixture of paraffin and vaselin, employing the same technique as previously described, except that the paraffin should have a melting point slightly above the normal temperature of the body, between 99 and 100° F. Injected beneath the mucous membrane lining the alveolar sockets of teeth, immediately after their extraction and the stoppage of hemorrage, it will prevent the entire absorption of the bone. This is of great importance, especially in the preservation of the cuspid eminence, retaining the facial contour; and in cases where all the teeth have been removed and artificial dentures are to be substituted, the cuspid eminence will form the foundation for the setting up of artificial teeth.

Gersuny reports a number of cases in which he substituted paraffin for absent parts, and since his publication other well known surgeons have employed his treatment in pathological conditions of like character. Dr. Maszkowicz (*Wiener Klinische Wochenschrift*, 1901, No. 25) reports the injection of paraffin about the ends of a resected nerve, to prevent their union; also the introduction of paraffin between the joint after the breaking of an old ankylosis, to prevent recurrence of adhesions. A small opening between the nose and the mouth, left after staphylorrhaphy, was closed by paraffin. The best results in this treatment are obtained in the correction of deformities following cicatricial contractions from loss of tissue through disease or operative procedure. Last September I injected paraffin into the alveloar sockets of the upper cuspids. The opening became occluded with granulation tissue; and a few weeks ago, when I last saw the patient, a decided prominence was noticeable where the paraffiu injection was made. Dr. RUDOLPH BECK, in *Dental Digest.—Dental Era.*

Dental Clippings.

To Contributors and Correspondents.

Original articles, clinical reports, correspondence upon subjects of general or special interest, news items, etc., are solicited from members of the profession everywhere.

The editor is not responsible for the statements or opinions of contributors.

All communications for the editor, original contributions, exchanges, books for review, etc., should be addressed to DR. CHAS. H. EDGE, No. 308 and 309 Kiam Building, Houston Texas.

All communications of a business nature, all drafts, checks, money orders, etc., should be addressed and made payable to THE A. P. CARY Co., Publisher, Houston, Texas.

Subscription price, 50 cents per annum.

Editorial Department.

The Patent Bill May Become a Law During the Next Congress.

The prospects are now good for the passage of the Patent Bill at the next session of Congress. This bill has been "bobbing" up before the Patent Committee for the past few years, only to be pigeon-holed until more effort was spent by the Dental Societies of the country in inducing some one else to take it up. Not baffled by continual defeats, and with a strong determination to win, the leaders of this movement finally succeeded through the influence of Dr. Emory A. Bryant, of Washington, D. C., in interesting the Hon. Geo. W. Taylor, of Alabama. Mr. Taylor was so enthusiastic in his belief in the justice of such a law that he worked unceasingly with the members of the Patent Committee until, with a few changes in the wording of the original bill, it has been reported favorably, and is now on the calendar for passage during the next session.

The National Dental Association, at its recent meeting at Niagara Falls, appreciating the valuable services of the Hon. Mr. Taylor, unanimously adopted the following resolution:

WHEREAS, The National Dental Association, the representative body of American Dentists, being interested in House Bill, No. 12451, introduced by Mr. Geo. W. Taylor, of Alabama, and recognizing the able, zealous and untiring labor which the

Hon. Mr. Taylor has expended in gaining the unanimous approval of the bill by the Patent Committee of the House of Representatives;

Resolved, That the National Dental Association extends its heartfelt thanks to the Hon. Geo. W. Taylor, of Alabama.

Colorado State Board of Dental Examiners.

The Board of Dental Examiners of the State of Colorado, will meet in Denver, Colorado, Tuesday, December 2nd, 1902, at 9 a. m., for the examination of applicants for license to practice dentistry in Colorado.

In addition to written and oral examination, applicants must supply their own patients, instruments and materials, and come prepared to do practical work under the supervision of the Board, which will pass upon suitable selection of cavities.

All applications must be completed prior to December 2nd.

For application blanks and information, address

H. F. Hoffman, Secretary,
611 California Bld'g, Denver, Colo.

The International Dental Congress at St. Louis.

At the recent meeting at Niagara Falls, of the National Dental Association, a resolution was adopted inviting the Federation Dentarie Internationale to hold the fourth annual meeting in St. Louis in the month of August, 1904, during the Louisiana Purchase Exposition to be held in that city in spring, summer, and autumn of that year.

Drs. Eugene H. Smith, of Boston, Truman W. Brophy, of Chicago, and William C. Barrett, of Buffalo, were appointed commissioners to present the invitation to the International Federation at the meeting held in Stockholm, Sweden, in August last. The invitation thus officially extended was accepted by cable August 18th.

For the organization and conduct of this important meeting the President of the National Dental Association, Dr. J. A. Libby, appointed the following committee:

Dr. Edward C. Kirk, Philadelphia.

Dr. R. H. Hofheinz, Rochester, N. Y.

Dr. H. J. Burkhart, Batavia, N. Y.

Dr. Wm. Carr, New York.

Dr. Waldo E. Boardman, Boston.

Dr. V. E. Turner, Raleigh, N. C.

Dr. J. Y. Crawford, Nashville, Tenn.

Dr. M. F. Finley, Washington, D. C.

Dr. J. W. David, Corsicana, Tex.

Dr. Wm. Crenshaw, Atlanta, Ga.

Dr. Don M. Gallie, Chicago.

Dr. Geo. V. I. Brown, Milwaukee.

Dr. A. H. Peck, Chicago.

Dr. J. D. Patterson, Kansas City.

Dr. Burton Lee Thorpe, St. Louis.

A committee so representative and so capable can be safely trusted to make the Fourth International Dental Congress, what it doubtless will be, an event memorable in professional history, and of incalculable value in promoting professional interests and harmonizing professional relations throughout the world.— *Dental Brief.*

In Memoriam.

DR. H. A. DREWRY died, at the home of his son in Nacogdoches, Texas, on October 1, 1902, after an illness of short duration, caused principally by his old age.

Dr. Drewry was born in Forsythe, Georgia, April 3, 1826. He began the study and practice of dentistry in the office of Dr. Surcey, in Macon, Ga., in 1850. Remaining there four years, he removed to Tuscaloosa, Ala., where he practiced until 1860. He then came to Texas, and settled at Salem, Rusk county. In 1861 he volunteered his services to the Confederate cause. After having served two years in Walker's division, as a private, he was promoted to act as regimental dentist, which place he continued to fill until the close of the war, Returning after the war, he again took up the practice in the counties of Rusk, Cherokee and Shelby, and continued up to about six months before he died.

Dr. Drewry was married December 23, 1852, to Miss Sallie A. Thomas, at Griffin, Ga. His wife died August 2, 1882. From this happy union there came five children, three of them living —James A. Drewry, F. O. Drewry, and S. A. Drewry.

Dr. Drewry was a man of more than ordinary mechanical ability. Having had to work out for himself the intricate details of the foundation of our profession naturally developed his mind along those lines more than if he had had it given him by college professors. He was gentle and painstaking with his patients, ever mindful of his duty to them, and was highly esteemed throughout the circle of his acquaintance as a dutiful professional gentleman. He was probably the oldest dentist in Texas.

Recent Patents of Interest to Dentists.

706,710—Receptacle for tooth-powder or other material, Joseph C. Allen, Plainfield, N. J.

707,810—Dental form for holding teeth, Raymond J. Wenker, Milwaukee, Wis.

708,811—Machine for forcibly casting dental bridges, Merrill W. Hollingsworth, Philadelphia, Pa.

708,772—Dental-gold annealer, Chapin F. Lauderdale, Milwaukee, Wis.

709,410—Dental bridgework, John L. Kelly, St. Paul, Minn.

709,049—Machine for forming aud drying toothpicks, Charles F. Scamman, deceased, Portland, Me., T. L. Scamman, administratrix.

709,050—Machine for drying toothpicks, Charles F. Scamman, deceased, Portland, Me., T. L. Scamman, administratrix.

709,812—Dental mouth mirror, George S. Bennett, and J. W. Thatcher, San Francisco, Cal.

709,834—Dental gage, Clarence R. Vanderpool, Grand Rapids, Michigan.

709,973—Dental apparatus, Lucien Eilertsen, Paris, France.

709,927—Tooth brush and powder cabinet, Corwin T. Price, Washington, D. C.

710,306—Rubber dam﹐holder, George W. Todd, Elmwood, Omaha, Nebr.

710,444—Means for attaching tooth members, Willis H. Dwight, Lemars, Iowa.

710,498—Toothpick, Dow McClain, Kansas City, Kans.

710,638—Dental cuspidor, Joseph E. Van Nostran, Canton, Ohio.

Soldering Hint.

BY L. C. TAYLOR, D. D. S., HARTFORD, CONN.

When soldering crowns or bridges requiring a number of pieces of solder, first pickle well in acid so surfaces will be bright, then place solder in quantity about as needed, drop a few drops of sticky wax on it to hold solder in place, put borax over the wax, and heat up slowly to dry out. Then with blow-pipe bring the mass to a white heat, allowing the wax to burn out, and see how quickly the work will be completed without the solder crawling with borax or dropping from some slight jar of the case. The solder for a full plate can be put in place when plate is cold under the above method with great satisfaction. It has been suggested that the borax would flow with the wax, soak into investment, and crack the porcelain, but I have soldered with this method for more than a year and have never had a porcelain crack. Several friends to whom I have suggested this plan report that they are employing it all the time with gratifying results.—*Dental Digest.*

Time to Laugh.

Dr. Herbert W. Spencer tells the following story of his attempt to corner a Christian Scientist:

"Every time we met, this Scientist took occasion to scoff at medical practice and to dwell upon the wonders which could be performed through faith. 'You are convinced that through faith you can do anything?' I said to him one day.

"'Yes,' he replied, 'faith will move mountains.'

"A week later he was in my office with a swollen jaw due to a toothache. 'What, you here!' I exclaimed, with feigned astonishment.

"'Oh, doctor,' he said, 'I have suffered agony all through the night. I simply can't stand this pain any longer.'

"'Have you tried faith?' I said to him. 'You know you told me the other day that faith could move mountains.'

"'But this is a cavity, doctor; this is a cavity.'"—*New York Times.*

Have You Sent for Our New Catalogue of... Porcelain Teeth?

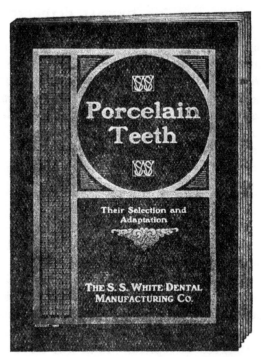

IT'S fresh from the printer, a volume of 187 pages, 7½x10 inches, and chock-full of meat for the prosthetic dentist.

It illustrates our line of molds of Porcelain Teeth, and it tells how to select and adapt, —how to utilize these molds to the best advantage.

Our line of molds is unequaled in its extent and variety. They represent the forms and sizes of the Porcelain Teeth which are universally known to be superior in their combination of the essential qualities,—naturalness of appearance, strength, adaptability, and ease of manipulation.

The prosthetic dentist who is not in touch with our stock of Porcelain Teeth, with its unapproached facilities for selection, fails to realize the possibilities of his art. This Catalogue will put you in touch with it. The cost to you will be a postal card request. Send for it now.

THE S. S. WHITE DENTAL MFG. CO.,

Philadelphia, New York. Boston, Chicago, Brooklyn, Atlanta, Rochester, Berlin, Buenos Aires. St. Petersburg, Toronto.

Dental Floss Silk

Thinness and Strength.

From the nature of its uses, Floss Silk must possess two attributes, without which it will be valueless to the dentist and its use an annoying hindrance instead of a help. It must be thin and it must be strong. It is easy to get the thinness, the fineness of the silk fiber lending itself to any degree of tenuity. The strength is not so easy. While silk filament is of itself strong, the maker of Dental Floss Silk does not have the opportunity to increase this which is to be gained by twisting, as in making thread. The very idea of Floss Silk conveys the thought of softness, fluffiness. The tensile strength of Dental Floss Silk must depend upon the quality of the silk and the skill of the manufacturer in conserving the inherent strength of the fiber.

Pure, Uniform.

It is just in this essential of strength that our Dental Floss Silk excels. The stock used is the best Japanese and Chinese. The treatment throughout the process of manufacture is directed to the conservation and concentration of strength. There is on adulteration of any kind, nor is there any dye-stuff used, to the possible disintegration of the fiber, or that might cause an unpleasant taste in the mouth. The finished product—the plain variety—is silk, and nothing but silk. (The waxed has only the wax, which is of the finest quality white wax and is strictly pure, added for the easier placing in narrow spaces.) It is free from knots and inequalities, is uniform throughout. It has the highest degree of tensile strength known to products of its character. It would hardly serve to weigh the anchor of an ocean liner, but it will stand the strain of tying knots in ligatures. Every lot of it is tested before it goes into stock.

How Its Use Increases.

Our Dental Floss Silk has been before the profession for many years, and complaint as to its quality is unknown. What this means may perhaps be more clearly understood when it is considered that our business in it has grown so that it is to be computed by the 100,000 spools. It would be reckoned by the 1,000,000 if ever possible user were familiar with its superiority. It is unquestionably the best Floss Silk at the service of dentists and for personal use.

Plain and Waxed, put up in

12-Yard, 24-Yard, and 150-Yard Spools.

PRICES.

			Per gross.	Per half-gross.	Per dozen.	Per spool.
Plain.	12 yd.	(Black Boxes)	$7.00	$3.75	$0.75	$0.08
	24 "	Red "		6.25	1.35	.15
	150 "	Black "		38.25	8.00	.75
Waxed.	12 "	" "	9.50	5.00	1.00	.10
	24 "	Red "		9.50	2.00	.20
	150 "	Black "		45.50	9.50	.90

The Waxed is also supplied in 6-yard Spools, just the right size for refilling our Floss Silk Holders.

	Per half-gross.	Per dozen.	Per spool.
Price, Waxed, 6-yard Spools	$3.00	$0.60	$0.06

THE S. S. WHITE DENTAL MFG. CO.,

Philadelphia, New York, Boston, Chicago, Brooklyn, Atlanta, Rochester, Berlin, Buenos Aires, St. Petersburg, Toronto.

THE S. S. WHITE DENTAL MFG. CO.'S

TRADE

Dental Base ⚭ Plate Rubbers.

MARK

Our new line of Dental Base-Plate Rubbers includes all the accepted shades:

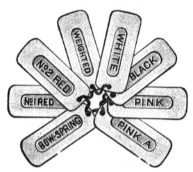

Bow-Spring.	A medium brown.
No. 1 Red.	A reddish brown, lighter than the Bow-Spring.
No. 2 Red.	A still lighter shade.
Weighted.	A mottled red, for lower cases.
Black.	A clear jet black.
White.	A light drab, approaching white, for veneering.
Pink.	A dark pinkish tint, for veneering.
Pink A.	A lighter pink, for veneering.

Bow-Spring, No. 1 Red, No. 2 Red. Weighted, and Black are the regular Base-Plate brands, the Weighted for lower dentures specially. White, Pink, and Pink A are intended for facing or veneering plates made of the regular Base-Plate brands.

Everybody knows the superior quality of our Bow-Spring Rubber. We have improved it, making it softer and easier to manipulate. All the others are of the same standard.

Our Dental Base-Plate Rubbers are pure, they are clean, they work easily, they are full weight. Any of our regular Base-Plate brands will make a strong, durable, satisfactory plate.

PRICES:

Bow-Spring No. 1 Red No. 2 Red Weighted Black }	.... {	per pound, $2.00 5 pound lots, " " 1.80 25 " " " " 1.70
White, for veneering) Pink " " Pink A, " " }	.... {	per pound, $3.00 5 pound lots, " " 2.70 25 " " " " 2.55

Put up in half-pound boxes.

For Testing Purposes.

We want every dentist to test these Rubbers practically. To this end we put up a sample box, containing a full sheet of each of the eight brands, together with a set of samples showing how each of them vulcanizes.

Price, sample box.....................................$1.00

THE S. S. WHITE DENTAL MFG. CO.,

Philadelphia, New York, Boston, Chicago, Brooklyn, Atlanta, Rochester, Berlin
Buenos Aires, St. Petersburg, Toronto.

Lightning Source UK Ltd.
Milton Keynes UK
UKHW012329061118
331891UK00010B/1028/P